No Longer Afraid of the Big, Bad Wolf

Dene' Danielle Hopkins

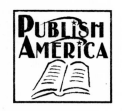

PublishAmerica

Baltimore

First printing

ISBN: 1-4137-0868-4
PUBLISHED BY PUBLISHAMERICA, LLLP
www.publishamerica.com
Baltimore

Printed in the United States of America

This book is dedicated to my husband Tom, who still makes my heart skip a beat, and to my children, Stephen, who always makes me laugh, and Courtney, who always takes my side. I love you all

SLOW ME DOWN, LORD

Slow me down, Lord
Ease the pounding of my heart
by the quieting of my mind.
Steady my hurried pace with a vision
of the eternal reach of time.
Give me, amid the confusion of the day,
the calmness of the everlasting hills.
Break the tensions of my nerves and
muscles with the soothing music of the
singing streams that live in my memory.
Help me to know the magical, restoring
power of sleep.
Teach me the art of taking minute vacations,
of slowing down to look at a flower, to chat
with a friend, to pat a dog, to read a few
lines from a good book.
Slow me down, Lord, and inspire me to
send my roots deep into the soil of life's
enduring values that I may grow
toward the stars of my greater destiny.

Chapter 1

Living the fairy tale

"Come and sit down beside my bed, dearie," wheezed the Wolf, "and let us have a little chat." Then the Wolf stretched out his large hairy paws and began to unfasten the basket.

"Oh!" said Red Riding-Hood, "what great arms you have, Grannie!"

"All the better to hug you with," said the Wolf.

"And what great rough ears you have, Grannie!"

"All the better to hear you with, my little dear."

"And your eyes, Grannie; what great yellow eyes you have!"

"All the better to see you with, my pet," grinned the Wolf.

"And oh! oh! Grannie," cried the child, in a sad fright, "what great sharp teeth you have!"

"All the better to eat you with!" growled the Wolf, springing up suddenly at Red Riding-Hood.

In a sense, I *was* Red Riding Hood. I had lived a fairy tale life complete with marriage to a prince and happily ever after. Nothing in life had really been difficult for me - until then. I had been a good student with lots of friends and had married a wonderful Christian man with whom I was raising two incredible children. Marriage and parenting weren't necessarily a piece of cake, but compared to some, mine were relatively easy to handle. But the wolf I encountered that day on my path through life was soon to take on a life of its own by becoming a very unwelcome member of our family.

Although it may sound strange to compare a debilitating disease to a member of the family, that's the only way I know how to describe it. Haven't you ever heard the phrase, "You can pick your friends, but you can't pick your family?" We aren't born with much say in the matter as to who our parents are, let alone embracing cousin Shirley, who has more facial hair than most men and drives a John Deere riding mower to the grocery store!

The doctor didn't say to me that spring day, "So, what disease would you like to test drive? Would you like the super dooper heart attack that could get you to heaven nice and fast? Or maybe you prefer cancer, a disease that is a bit slower than a heart attack, which gives you more opportunity to enjoy the important things in life, but takes away your dignity in the process as you lose your hair, not to mention the friends who can't handle being around someone who already has one foot in the grave? But at least people will recognize it from the name alone, maybe even having a family member who took the cancer test drive. Better yet, why not try out this slow, painful one that no one understands or even tries to? Then you will be all alone in your final journey, with few who can sympathize, knowing little to nothing about it, but many who will speculate as to how well you must be handling the ride, since you certainly look so good doing it?"

Chapter 2

Looking good in the red cape

About the only value the story of my life may have is to show that one can, even without any particular gifts, overcome obstacles that seem insurmountable if one is willing to face the fact that they must be overcome. -- Eleanor Roosevelt

If I've heard it once, I've heard it a dozen times. People approach me and question me as to how I'm feeling. Perhaps I've had to be home, unable to really get out and socialize, and they, knowing I've been sick, inquire as to how I'm doing. I can usually tell by the look in their eyes that they have some doubt, especially if I happen to be having a good hair day and have managed to successfully cover the circles under my eyes. Of course some people simply use the phrase "How are you doing?" in place of hello, and don't *really* want to know the gory details, and to those I simply reply "fine" and go on, as we all do. But then there are those who are curious and a little judgmental, who base their conclusion of how sick someone is by their own experience, which usually consists of an occasional stomach virus and the yearly cold. They know that when they spend a day or two hugging the toilet, the last thing they are concerned with is their physical appearance! So how can someone who is noticeably absent more than she is present look so normal?

I've often wondered just what those people *expect* to see. I think I have an idea. They expect me to stumble about, clutching my terry cloth robe so as not to expose the oversized stained nightshirt underneath, wearing house slippers and tube socks, not having brushed my hair in days, no make-up and nothing but a sour expression on my face! Not to say that I don't have those days, I do, we all do. Having a chronic illness changes many, many things, both physically and emotionally. But it doesn't change who I am! I am still a child of God, full of the life He gave me.

I am still the person who loves to laugh at my husband's corny

9

jokes. I am still the mother who waits anxiously for her children to walk in the door after school just to be able to listen to them squabble with each other over whose turn it is to empty the dishwasher. I am the person who wants to get invited to lunch with the ladies, in spite of the fact that I probably will not be able to go. I am still the church member who, although unable to worship standing next to you, is worshipping at home, singing at the top of my lungs and lifting my hands in praise. I am the daughter who wants to be included in the typical family gatherings and asked to bring a covered dish, but forgiven when that's not possible and all I can provide is a smile. I am the person who tries to find the good in every day, in spite of how I feel. I am the woman who, on those bad days, finds a little joy in being able to make it to the front window to watch the birds gather twigs to build their home in hopes of filling it with little blue speckled eggs. And I am the woman who savors every minute that God gives me, not just the minutes that are without pain, but especially the ones that cause me to cry out to Him. For in pain, I am reminded of just how much He loves me, for He suffered too.

I am not alone. The Lupus Foundation of America (www.lupus.org) estimates that 1.4 million Americans suffer from some form of Lupus, and that 9 out of 10 are women. Lupus is now listed as a leading cause of morbidity among women, and that women are 5 times more likely to die from complications of Lupus than were men.

Even though I may feel lousy on the inside, the last thing I want to do is *look* lousy, too. God knows I look at myself in the mirror day after day and see a face that is not just aging, but feeling the effects of disease. And I don't even bother looking at the rest of my body in the mirror! I've long since lost my waistline, and my boobs are sagging so low, I now have a combination going I refer to as my baistline.

So, of course, I'm going to do my best to cover that up when I go out. I've become a master of disguise in a way, which is part of the reason behind this book. To uncover the truth behind this disease and to give healthy, normal people a look into the lives of families afflicted with chronic illnesses. The intention is not just to allow you a peek into only my life, but the lives of those who have to carry the burden as caregivers.

In order to fully understand the dynamics of the family with chronic disease, I will also introduce you to a few members of the wolf family, hopefully giving you an even better glimpse into our lives.

Mostly, I want you the reader to *empathize* with those of us with chronic illness. I am not looking for, nor do I need sympathy. But the missing link in the battle to live with this affliction is people who cannot and refuse to identify with their friends and co-workers with Lupus. Hopefully, after reading this book, your shoes will be completely stretched out from walking several miles in mine.

Chapter 3

Meeting the Wolf

If you want to live a long life, get a chronic disease and learn how to take care of it. -- Sir William Osler

The day began like every other day. It was the spring of 1993, and I was working as a teacher's aide at an elementary school in Moore, Oklahoma. My job wasn't the typical aide position, running copies and grading papers. Surprisingly, my job was stressful and complicated by the fact that the students I assisted were not the "normal" students, but were labeled "EMR" – educable mentally retarded. My students looked just like every other student. Their speech wasn't slurred, and their socio-economic backgrounds varied as in most public school settings. What made my kids different were several factors. Their social behavior and ability to adapt to their peers played a large part, coupled with their IQ, which ranged from 75 to 90. That's why they were considered educable. Their limitations were not so severe that they would never be able to function as a contributing member of society, rather that they could be taught, if given the appropriate time and methods.

Looking back, it's really a little ironic. I was in a position to not only nurture and assist those who needed special care, but also to defend and protect them. We've all heard it said that children can, at times, be cruel. I'd like to believe the cruelty, the name-calling, the prejudice all stems from immaturity and ignorance, but unfortunately that is not always the case. Spend a few minutes with a parent of a kid who calls names, and you'll find someone who judges and excludes others with differences. Don't get me wrong, these rules do not always apply, but more often than not, they do.

Many times throughout my days at work, especially on days when I had playground duty, I found myself coming to the defense of the kids in my class. Sometimes it was for being called a retard or hurt feelings from being excluded in a game, but mostly from just plain ignorance.

Early on, society teaches our children what normal looks like. If someone doesn't fit into that description, even though their physical appearance looks quite ordinary, society tells us to keep our distance, to shy away from and to stick to those who are more like us. The world doesn't encourage us to accept those who are different than us.

I could write an entire book just on the prejudices and judgments that occur throughout our lives, but that's not the point. The point I am trying to make is that, just like the kids in my class who were judged harshly because their outside didn't match their inside, I can look just like you on the outside, and yet be racked by pain on the inside with every breath I take, and no one would ever be able to tell.

I say that not to sound pious or to boast, but to emphasize the fact that my demeanor is a *CHOICE*. My personality doesn't change just because of a disease. Both my father and my stepmother taught me great lessons in the area of behavior when sick. Although my dad's line was always "be tough," he also taught me not to complain or focus on the pain or sickness. If I had a stomachache, I would hold my stomach, the natural reaction to pain. But if he saw me doing this, he would frown at me and instruct me to quit holding my stomach and stand up straight. At the time, being a normal kid, I just thought he was being insensitive, when instead the bigger lesson was that when we're hurting, taking the focus mentally off the pain can lesson and even make the pain tolerable.

Learning a similar life lesson from my stepmother came one day shortly after experiencing the monthly *joy* of being a woman. I awakened with cramps, and not having experienced them before, fully intended to stay in bed until they left. But she quickly pointed out to me that this blessed event would barge into my life every month for the next 40 years, and that the world won't stop just because I'm hormonal. She explained to me that laundry would still need to be washed, meals would still need to be cooked, my husband and children would still need tending to, and I needed to learn early that life goes on whether you're in pain or you're not. Again, I wasn't too thrilled with her lesson and would have preferred a little sympathy for my monthly condition, but none was to be had. Several years later I would hear myself repeating those same wise words to my daughter, not to be insensitive, but to teach her to cope with and prepare for the certainty that there would be pain on a regular, monthly basis.

On that day at my job in the school, when the pain began, I did like I had been taught and simply toughed it out. I had been tired and achy off and on for several months, but figured it was simply the changes we had been through the past several months. We had recently moved back to Oklahoma from Texas and were in the middle of having a home built, a stressful venture in itself. Not to mention the fact that I had gone back to work for the first time in several years in order to have a nice down payment for that home. I had also toughed it out through a recent bout of mononucleosis, but had not been able to take the time off to fully recuperate. I had gone to work every day in spite of feeling extreme fatigue and pounding headaches. But by the time lunch rolled around, the Tylenol I had taken still hadn't taken worked, and naturally, I had playground duty.

We hadn't been back in the classroom long when I noticed a tingly feeling in both of my feet, almost like the feeling you get when a body part goes to "sleep". Before long it had traveled up my legs to my knees and thighs, along with some swelling, and within an hour I was nearly unable to walk. The swelling was so apparent that the other teacher noticed it before I even had a chance to tell her. She encouraged me to go ahead and leave early. The next day was the beginning of a long weekend, and it would be difficult to get in to see a doctor.

By the time I got home, I could barely move. The swelling had continued up my body and a rash had developed. The only thing I could do was lay down, since the swelling made it difficult to sit. My joints were unable to bend under the pressure of the fluid I was retaining.

The normal person would do the natural thing and call the doctor or even perhaps go to the emergency room. For reasons I still don't understand to this day, I made the decision to stay home and hope that it would go away. It wasn't that I was trying to be tough or cope with the pain as I had been taught, it was more a matter of ignorance, plus the fact that it was now past 5 p.m. and the following day was a three-day holiday weekend. I guess I just figured that if it were still a problem after the weekend, then I would go. It really never occurred to me to go to the ER, even though the swelling was making it difficult to breathe, and the rash had begun to itch terribly. Looking back, it was probably the grace of God that kept me alive that weekend. The swelling was even causing my kidneys to stop functioning, and although I was extremely thirsty and drinking constantly, I didn't go to the bathroom more than one or two times the entire weekend.

By Monday, the swelling was going down, and the rash was gone. In its place came achy and tender muscles and joints. I managed to drag myself to work, but over the course of the next few days as the swelling went away, the joint pain increased. The teacher I worked with was completely baffled as to why I hadn't gone to the doctor. She not only insisted that I go see one, she even made me an appointment herself with an Internist.

The doctor was a small woman with an energy that implied impatience and busyness, and after questioning me about the incident, appeared very frustrated with me. She came across as though she thought I was ignorant for not going to the ER. She informed me first that I was overweight, a statement I was just thrilled to hear. Obviously, she wasn't concerned about making friends with me! She then began a barrage of questions about my personal life, what I liked to do in my free time, if I had any hobbies, etc. Now I was frustrated, since I simply wanted a quick fix for whatever was wrong with me, a prescription or just a simple diagnosis would have been fine. Appearing not to like my answers, she made several marks on my chart, and I felt like I was in trouble, like I had done something wrong. Insisting that I was experiencing stress, she kept repeating to me that I needed to reduce it, but not knowing the effect that stress could have on health, I turned a deaf ear, ignoring her suggestions.

She didn't give me a diagnosis, but instead quickly listed several things that could be the problem, most of which I had never heard of. The only one that I even remotely understood was Rheumatoid Arthritis. A friend of my grandmother's had RA and suffered with a lot of pain. She also had what I considered to be deformities of her hands and feet caused by the RA.

Finished with questioning me and ready to go on to her next patient, she sent me to the lab for blood work and x-rays. The nurse told me that they would call me sometime in the next couple of weeks to let me know the results, and then promptly requested a check to pay for the appointment in the amount of $350! And before I could catch my breath from the shock, she quickly informed me that I would also be getting a bill for the lab work. Talk about confusing! First she wants me to reduce the stress in my life, and then she stresses me out by charging me a fortune to be mean to me!

The next couple of weeks passed in a blur, and even though I was in constant pain, I continued to do all the things I had always done. When the call finally came from the doctor's office, I was surprised to find the doctor herself at the other end of the line. Hoping and praying for anything but Rheumatoid Arthritis, I was relieved when she told me that I most likely had Systemic Lupus. She mentioned something about having 8 of the 11 symptoms, along with a positive ANA. She might as well have been speaking French, because it was all foreign to me. Therefore, I didn't question her about what I should do, and although I am sure she suggested I make an appointment to see her again, I knew that I could never afford to go back with prices like that. I was only making a little over $7 an hour at the time, and her office fee was more than I earned in two weeks. Besides, I was so happy that I didn't have RA, I hung up and felt a big sense of relief.

It was back to work as usual the following day, and when my co-workers asked me what the diagnosis was, I happily replied that it was just Lupus. Most of them seemed just as relieved as I; none of them knew what it was either. But when the teacher I worked with heard me say that I had Systemic Lupus, she got this look on her face, not one of relief and joy like everyone else had, but more of disappointment. Sensing that I was completely clueless, as I was, she encouraged me to go to the library and do some research.

I suppose that was when the denial set in. First of all, there was very little information about Lupus to be found, and what information I could find, I somehow managed to convince myself didn't apply to me. Figuring that if I didn't acknowledge or believe the doctor's diagnosis, it would somehow go away. That stage of denial would last for over 6 years, costing me in more ways than I could have ever imagined.

Chapter 4

Who is the Wolf?

Everyone has limits. You just have to learn what your own limits are and deal with them accordingly. -- Nolan Ryan, American Baseball Player

Lupus is Latin for wolf and is the term used in the formal names of different species of wolves. Some think that the butterfly-shaped facial rash that often accompanies the disease resembles the markings of a wolf, therefore the origin for the name of the disease, Lupus. Lupus is a chronic inflammatory disease that can affect various parts of the body, especially the skin, joints, blood and kidneys. The body's immune system normally makes proteins called antibodies to protect the body against viruses, bacteria and other foreign materials. These foreign materials are called antigens. In an autoimmune disorder such as lupus, the immune system loses its ability to tell the difference between foreign substances (antigens) and its own cells and tissues. The immune system then makes antibodies directed against self. These antibodies, called "auto-antibodies," react with the "self" antigens to form immune complexes. The immune complexes build up in the tissues and can cause inflammation, injury to tissues and pain. Think of it as a 'self-allergy' where the body attacks its own cells and tissues, causing inflammation, pain and possible organ damage.

For most people, lupus is a mild disease affecting only a few organs. For others, it may cause serious and even life-threatening problems. More than 16,000 Americans develop lupus each year. It is estimated that 500,000 to 1.5 million Americans have been diagnosed with lupus.

In simple words, when the normal person gets sick, their immune system fights it off. In a body affected by Lupus, the immune system doesn't know when to stop attacking. It attacks the healthy tissue, causing pain and swelling.

There are two main types of Lupus. *Discoid* Lupus is always limited to the skin. It is identified by a rash that may appear on the face, neck and scalp. Discoid lupus does not generally involve the body's internal organs. In approximately 10 percent of patients, discoid lupus can evolve into the systemic form of the disease, which can affect almost any organ or system of the body. This cannot be predicted or prevented. Treatment of discoid lupus will not prevent its progression to the systemic form. Individuals who progress to the systemic form probably had systemic lupus at the outset, with the discoid rash as their main symptom. *Systemic* lupus is usually more severe than discoid lupus and can affect almost any organ or system of the body. For some people, only the skin and joints will be involved. In others, the joints, lungs, kidneys, blood, other organs and/or tissues may be affected. Generally, no two people with systemic lupus will have identical symptoms. Systemic lupus may include periods in which few, if any, symptoms are evident ("remission") and other times when the disease becomes more active ("flare"). Most often when people mention "lupus," they are referring to the systemic form of the disease.

Flares (What triggers lupus)

What triggers an attack of lupus in a susceptible person? Scientists have noted common features in many lupus patients. In some, exposure to the sun causes sudden development of a rash and then possibly other symptoms. In others an infection, perhaps a cold or a more serious infection, does not get better and then complications arise. These complications may be the first signs of lupus. In still other cases, a drug taken for some illness produces the signaling symptoms. In some women, the first symptoms and signs develop during pregnancy. In others, they appear soon after delivery. Many people cannot remember or identify any specific factor. Obviously, many seemingly unrelated factors can trigger the onset of the disease.

Over the years, in spite of the outward appearance of my denial and the inner turmoil of acceptance, I've learned to identify the things that cause flares for me. Stress was probably the most common trigger in the early years, or rather the inability to manage the stress. Denial played a huge part in keeping me from taking the proper care of myself, so instead of resting when I was tired or learning to say no to numerous activities, projects, etc., I just pushed myself even harder. I would push myself for several days or even weeks at a time with little to no breaks. My body would then crash, refusing to do anything, which resulted in several days in bed.

I also felt very guilty, as though I was somehow at fault. Mostly I felt guilt because I could no longer do everything I wanted to do with my kids, missing out on family bike rides because my knees were swollen or having to stay home while everyone else went to church. At the time, I thought other people made me feel guilty due to their questions about my lack of attendance at every church function or their comments about how I didn't *look* sick. Now I know that no one makes you feel guilty, that those feelings are self-imposed, and the guilt I felt at that time was probably due to my own denial and ignorance.

Cause

The cause(s) of lupus is unknown, but there are environmental and genetic factors involved. While scientists believe there is a genetic predisposition to the disease, it is known that environmental factors also play a critical role in triggering lupus. Some of the environmental factors that may trigger the disease are: infections, antibiotics (especially those in the sulfa and penicillin groups), ultraviolet light, extreme stress, certain drugs and hormones.

Although lupus is known to occur within families, there is no known gene or genes that are thought to cause the illness. There are recent discoveries of a gene on chromosome 1, which is associated with lupus in certain families. Previously, genes on chromosome 6 called "immune response genes" were also associated with the disease. Only 10 percent of lupus patients will have a close relative (parent or sibling) who already has or may develop lupus. Statistics show that only about 5% of the children born to individuals with lupus will develop the illness.

Lupus is often called a "woman's disease" despite the fact that many men are affected. Lupus can occur at any age and in either sex, although it occurs 10-15 times more frequently among adult females than among adult males after puberty or after the emergence into sexual maturity. The symptoms of the disease are the same in men and women. People of African, American Indian, and Asian origin are thought to develop the disease more frequently than Caucasian women. The reasons for this ethnic selection are not clear.

Hormonal factors may explain why lupus occurs more frequently in females than in males. The increase of disease symptoms before menstrual periods and/or during pregnancy support the belief that hormones, particularly estrogen, may somewhat regulate the way the disease progresses. However, the exact reason for the greater prevalence of lupus in women is unknown.

Treatment

For the vast majority of people with lupus, effective treatment can minimize symptoms, reduce inflammation and maintain normal bodily functions.

Preventive measures can reduce the risk of flares. For photosensitive patients, avoidance of excessive sun exposure and/or the regular application of sunscreens will usually prevent rashes. Regular exercise helps prevent muscle weakness and fatigue. Talking with support groups, counseling, family members, friends and physicians can help alleviate the effects of stress. Needless to say, negative habits are hazardous to people with lupus. These include smoking, excessive consumption of alcohol, too much or too little of prescribed medication or postponing regular medical checkups. By staying in a state of denial, I seldom saw a doctor, and when I did, I saw my family doctor, who treated me as best he could, but could only treat the symptoms, not the causes. By not finding and seeing a specialist, my family doctor's treatment was like applying a band-aid to a severed artery.

Medications are often prescribed for people with lupus, depending on which organ(s) are involved and the severity of involvement. Effective patient-physician discussions regarding the selection of medication, its possible side effects and any changes in doses are vital. Commonly prescribed medications include Non-steroidal Anti-inflammatory Drugs (NSAIDs), including ibuprofen, naproxen and a large number of others.

Steroids are also a common medication, the most common being Prednisone. Because steroids have a variety of side effects, the dose has to be regulated to maximize the beneficial anti-immune/anti-inflammatory effects and minimize the negative side effects. Side effects occur more frequently when steroids are taken over long periods of time at high doses (for example, 60 milligrams of Prednisone taken daily for periods of more than one month). Such side effects include weight gain, a round face, acne, easy bruising, "thinning" of the bones (osteoporosis), high blood pressure, cataracts, onset of diabetes, increased risk of infection, stomach ulcers, hyperactivity and an increase of appetite.

Antimalarials, including Plaquenil, commonly used in the treatment of malaria, may also be very useful in some individuals with lupus. They are most often prescribed for skin and joint symptoms of lupus. It may take months before these drugs demonstrate a beneficial effect. Side effects are rare and consist of occasional diarrhea or rashes. Some antimalarial drugs can affect the eyes.

Immunomodulating drugs like Imuran and Cytoxan are in a group of agents known as cytotoxic or immunosuppressive drugs. These drugs act in a similar manner to the corticosteroid drugs, in that they suppress inflammation and tend to suppress the immune system. The side effects of these drugs include anemia, low white blood cell count and increased risk of infection. Their use may also predispose an individual to developing cancer later in life.

People with lupus should learn to recognize early symptoms of disease activity. That way they can help the physician know when a change in therapy is needed. Regular monitoring of the disease by laboratory tests can be valuable because noticeable symptoms may occur only after the disease has significantly flared. Changes in blood test results may indicate the disease is becoming active even before the patient develops symptoms of a flare. Generally, it seems that the earlier such flares are detected, the more easily they can be controlled. Also, early treatment may decrease the chance of permanent tissue or organ damage and reduce the time one must remain on high doses of drugs.

The hardest thing about the drugs used to treat Lupus is the fact that so many have such damaging side effects, some of which are worse than the disease itself. Some of the drugs I've taken over the course of the years have caused my hair to fall out in clumps; I've had weight gains and weight losses, nausea when exposed to light and rashes, just to name a few lovely side effects.

Symptoms of Lupus

Although lupus can affect any part of the body, most people experience symptoms in only a few organs. The most common symptoms of people with lupus are:

Achy joints	Skin rashes
Fever	Anemia
Arthritis (swollen joints)	Kidney involvement
Prolonged or extreme fatigue	Hair loss
Sun or light sensitivity	Butterfly
Abnormal blood clotting problems	
Pain in the chest while breathing deep/pleurisy	

Prognosis

The idea that lupus is generally a fatal disease is one of the gravest misconceptions about this illness. In fact, the prognosis of lupus is much better today than ever before.

It is true that medical science has not yet developed a method for curing lupus, and some people do die from the disease. However, people with non-organ threatening Lupus can look forward to a normal lifespan if they follow the instructions of their physician, take their medication(s) as prescribed and know when to seek help for unexpected side effects of a medication or a new manifestation of their lupus.

Although some people with lupus have severe recurrent attacks and are frequently hospitalized, most people with lupus rarely require hospitalization. There are many lupus patients who never have to be hospitalized, especially if they are careful and follow their physician's instructions.

New research brings unexpected findings each year. The progress made in treatment and diagnosis during the last decade has been greater than that made over the past 100 years. It is therefore a sensible idea to maintain control of a disease that tomorrow may be curable.

The denial years probably cost me since I rarely saw a doctor, and when I did, it was only when I was past the point where medical intervention would have prevented it to get so bad.

Going to the doctor is something I do not like to do. It's nothing personal against my doctors, most of the time they are wonderful, caring individuals. The main reason I avoid going to the doctor has to do with my personality. I don't like to complain, which keeps me from telling the doctor everything he or she needs to know, and I hate to ask for help.

But I'm doing better. I'm probably always going to be in denial, but I call it hope. Hope that someday soon there will be a cure, hope that someday God will heal me, hope that I won't give in and let Lupus win.

Denial's not so bad.

Chapter 5

"Good Morning, Mr. Wolf"

Laughter can draw others to you and lighten your load in life. When you begin to laugh at life and at yourself, you gain new perspectives on your struggle. Begin today. -- Emilie Barnes

How different our lives are when we really know what is deeply important to us, and keeping that picture in mind, we manage ourselves each day to be and to do what really matters most. -- Stephen Covey, American Speaker, Trainer, Author of "The 7 Habits of Highly Effective People"

Lupus affects each person differently and the symptoms, or flares, are dependent sometimes on what stage of Lupus the person is in or even how long they've been battling the disease.

When I was first diagnosed, I was in so much denial that instead of listening to my body when it needed to rest, I just pushed it harder, maybe in a way to prove to myself that I wasn't really sick. Besides the fact that I was dealing with a debilitating illness, I was still living the "people pleaser, do what is expected of me" lifestyle. I was so busy keeping everyone else happy and doing all the things that were expected of me, especially as a pastor's wife, that I was taking years off my life.

In the early years of this disease, the flares I experienced usually involved my joints. Every morning (and to this day), when I first placed my feet on the floor, there was immediate pain. In the beginning I used to wonder if I could ever live with this kind of ongoing pain, but it has become something I am used to. The only way to explain it is to use the analogy of being pinched. When someone pinches you, it hurts, but if they keep pinching you with the same amount of pressure, you eventually get used to it, and you adjust. The pain doesn't go away; it just becomes part of who you are.

As I mentioned, the pain was mostly in my joints, especially my knees and hips. I could be walking just fine one minute, and the next be consumed with pain so severe that I couldn't put one foot in front of the other. At times Lupus would attack with a vengeance, causing swelling around the knee, making it impossible to walk without crutches. And just as mysteriously as it would appear, it would disappear. Usually the flares happened right before one big event or right after. My husband and I even got to the point that we expected and planned for the flares, obviously always hopeful that they wouldn't happen, but prepared just the same.

Lupus has affected my knees, ankles, toes, fingers, wrists, elbows, hips, shoulders and ribs. I have had steroid injections in my knees more times than I can count and injections in my chest where my ribs connect to my sternum. While Lupus continues to attack the joints of my body, it now has begun its attack on my organs. Lupus has attacked my kidneys, my stomach, my gall bladder, my esophagus and my lungs. The constant discomfort in my lungs is probably the most painful, since it hurts to breathe, and unfortunately, one has to breathe!

While Lupus has taken a huge toll on my body, it doesn't compare to the effect it has had on my life, that is, on my husband, my children and my friends. Lupus has made me a virtual prisoner in my home, keeping me from attending weddings, funerals, parties, church, awards ceremonies and sports events, just to name a few. Not only am I unable to be at different events and occasions, I am sometimes even judged by my peers and others for not being there. I have even been questioned by church members as to my whereabouts, even though they have been told that I have Lupus, but most are unwilling to accept Lupus as a valid excuse. I've often wondered if I had cancer, would I still get the same treatment? Probably not.

Lupus has affected my relationship with my husband the most. We are unable to make plans a lot of the time, because we don't know whether I am going to be able to participate. My husband has to carry a huge burden of not only caring for me, but also has to share the bulk of the household responsibilities that I normally would do. He has given up a lot to take care of me, and I am so grateful. It is very difficult not to feel guilty because of all that he has to do, and at times, it is hard for him to handle. He becomes angry for all that it robs us of, and I don't blame him. He isn't angry at me, rather at the disease, but I still feel responsible. Just in the few times that I've had to watch him struggle with his own pain after shoulder surgery or when he's been in bed with the flu, I hate the helpless feeling of not being able to make it better. It's difficult to see someone you love hurt, especially when you can't do anything to make it go away. I can't imagine what it's really like in the caregiver's shoes, especially for men, who, by nature, are the "fixers". Many husbands, unable to handle the huge burden of a lifelong debilitating disease, leave their wives. I thank God every day for sending me such a wonderful husband.

Instead of being angry or resentful, we have to be creative. Ordering dinner in, instead of going out for a special occasion, is one way. We rent movies and curl up in bed to watch them. Most importantly, we've learned to value the time we have and take advantage of the opportunities that come our way. We schedule occasional long weekends away at places that have amenities we both enjoy. But most importantly, we enjoy the moment. We spend more time making up when we disagree, instead of wasting time being angry. We've decided to pass on a legacy of love and patience to our children, showing them that when we stood before God and said our vows "for better and for worse, in sickness and in health", we meant it.

Lupus hasn't only had an effect on our personal life, but on our professional life as well. My husband has served in full time ministry since 1984, a profession that is far more stressful than most people realize. Studies show that many ministers will not live to see their 75th birthday. A couple of years ago, when I was at a stage in this disease that I wasn't sure I would even live through, we asked ourselves some hard questions that pertained to the church where my husband was serving as senior Pastor. The main question was this: If we could live anywhere, serve a church anywhere, have our children in school anywhere, where would it be? In addition to Lupus problems, we were experiencing tremendous pressure from that church, mostly I believe as a result of the Lupus. Most did not understand the disease, nor did they try to. Week after week when I would be asked how I was feeling, they would comment frequently that they didn't understand how I could have been so sick, when I looked just fine to them. At one point I was even accused of not liking the people since I wasn't in attendance much of the time. Did they honestly believe I was home eating bon bons and throwing parties on Sunday mornings? Did they think it was easy to see my children go to church without me, that I actually *liked* watching television evangelists? The pressure of pleasing them resulted in unbearable stress, and stress is a huge factor in Lupus flares. The more they pressured, the more stress they inflicted, the more I flared. The more I flared, the more I missed, the more they pressured. All a vicious cycle that was not to be resolved. We sought council and searched our hearts. We listened to what God had been trying to say to us for several months and left the position at the church, not sure of where we were going or what God had in store for us, but sure of our decision. Our family questioned us, our friends didn't understand, but we knew in our hearts we needed to be a part of a church family that embraced us and supported us. For the first time in our lives we had chosen to simply be members of a church family, to worship together. We were accepted by them as we were, without expectations. We were there because we had chosen to be there, and the feeling of being able to be ourselves was wonderful. When the decision was made to ask my husband to become part of the staff, the church already knew my limitations and accepted us anyway. The "expectation" burden has been lifted, and as a result, the stresses of ministry have been drastically lessened.

We have two children, two very active children, and they probably struggle with Lupus more than I will ever know. They are wonderful and supportive, but it does take a toll. I have had to miss out on everything from ballgames to awards assemblies, and I hate it. It's not only the big events, but even the family dinners when I've had to be in bed instead of sitting with them at the table, the bike rides, the hikes, the campouts; you name it, I've probably had to miss it at least once. They say children are resilient, that they are tough and adapt better than adults in difficult situations. While that may be true, no child enjoys having an ill parent. When my husband and I planned our family, we certainly didn't plan on Lupus invading our life. I never intended for my children to be raised by a sick mother.

My children are my priority, along with my husband, and the choices I make in order to be with them have cost me at times. But it is a price I'm willing to pay. It may cost me several days in bed because I've taken my daughter to a concert she wants to attend. Or it may cost me aches and pains because I've chosen to sit outside in freezing temperatures watching my son play baseball. At times it has cost me the opportunity to be a part of a Sunday morning worship service because I've chosen to spend Saturday shopping for school clothes. Unfortunately, some people don't agree with the choices I make. They don't understand that this disease doesn't allow me to do everything, that spending one day being where I need to be, where I want to be, involved in activity with my family, may mean that I can't be sitting in that pew on Sunday morning. But it doesn't ever mean that I don't want to be there.

Opportunities to spend time watching my son play golf or going to my daughter's band concerts will be over in a few years. By the time I am 43 years old, my children will both be out the door and enrolled in college, and the days spent shopping together or weekend movie marathons will be few and far between. I will have much more energy to put into being in church then, but for now, if I only have a few hours a week that are "good", my choice will always be that those hours belong to my family. Years from now it will not matter to them how many church functions I attended for the sake of the church people, but it will matter to them how I chose to spend my time, and that is the legacy that I must leave with them.

The effects of Lupus are both positive and negative, but the reality is that it is a part of my life, here to stay, at least for a while. That leaves me with a choice – I can be resentful, full of bitterness and walk around defeated, or I can hold my head up, smile and make the most of the gifts I have. My prayer is that Lupus will not define me, but will be just a part of who I am. When people are around me, I don't want them to immediately think of me as that woman who has a disease, but that they will think of me as that woman who smiles and laughs and makes other people feel good. I want them to see Jesus in me, not Lupus.

There's a song by Mary Mary called Shackles, and she sings about wanting the shackles off her feet so that she can dance, so she can praise. Lupus may be my shackles, but even it isn't strong enough to bind me and hold me back from anything, as long as Jesus holds the key. Even when I'm hurting, even when I can't find the strength to move, even when it may appear that Lupus has stolen my body, it will never own my heart.

Chapter 6

Living with the Wolf

The following are journal entries that are very personal, and yet need to be shared in order that you may see that I am human, but mostly you will see what living with Lupus is really like.

October, 1996
...Courtney wants me to come to the school to have lunch with her, but I am so fatigued that I can hardly breathe, let alone move. I hate to disappoint her, again, but how can I possibly be there. Not to mention, the pain in my hip is back, and it's causing me to limp. It's so embarrassing to have to limp – people stare at me, so it's easier to stay home than to have to endure the looks.

April, 1997
This is absolutely unbelievable! Of all weekends for this disease to show itself, it would have to be today. My knee started swelling around noon when I was packing, and now I can't bend my leg at all. We're leaving this evening for Muskogee to tryout at the church there, and the last thing I want them to see is me at my weakest.
...a full night of resting my leg has not made it better, it's worse now. The pain is almost more than I can stand, even with the pain pills the doctor called in for me. I didn't sleep at all. The swelling has moved into my hips, and not only could I not lay down because I couldn't get up if I needed to, but I can't find a comfortable position to even sit in.
...another night without sleep, and I'm so thirsty I can't stand it. Not only that, but no matter how much I drink, I haven't had to use the bathroom for almost 12 hours. I think I need to go to the ER, but Tom is so stressed. He's preaching in the morning and there is no way he can take me tonight. I called my parents, but how would it look if I'm not here in the morning? Lord, you're going to have to pull me through this one.

Although I made it through the flare prior to our move to Muskogee, Oklahoma, I continued to have small flares that just wouldn't leave me alone. But the summer of 2000 brought the beginning of one of the most difficult and longest flares yet. Instead of attacking my bones and joints, as was its custom, Lupus began attacking my lungs. At first the pain felt sharp, and I thought for a moment I may be having a heart attack. But the sharp pain subsided, leaving a constant dull pain in its place. This pain would last for almost 3 years.

August, 2000
...Another Sunday morning at home – I've finally stopped crying and feeling sorry for myself. What I would give to be able to go to church with my family! But I can't do everything. Each week I have to "choose" the activities I can participate in, and this week was particularly busy. School clothes shopping drained me for the rest of the week, but in order to be able to do that, I have to sacrifice something. I know people don't understand, especially church people.

They see me at the grocery store or the mall one day, but not at church the next. Do they honestly think I would choose to be home alone all the time?

September,, 2000
...I am going to die. I know I am dying, even though no one seems willing to talk about it. But aren't we all dying? Each day we live, we are closer, by one day, to the day we leave this life. The beauty of death overwhelms me. What a blessing and a joy to know that one's time is limited. My senses are heightened with every breath I draw, and I cannot seem to feel the skin of my husband enough. I lay my head on his chest and feel the rise and fall of his breathing, and I love him so much. He is so beautiful. I can only pray that he knows how much he means to me, because I do not have the words beyond I love you.

February, 2001
...I can count the number of close friends on one hand. Most of my friends give up after a while, and I can't blame them. I'm a terrible

friend. I used to make plans for lunch, always hopeful that I would be able to keep the appointment, but more often than not, I have to cancel. After a while, they just stop asking.

March, 2001

Lord, I pray for time. Time to watch my children grow into adulthood. Time to spend spoiling my grandkids. I long to see my children fulfill their dreams, to see the legacy unfold. I know how it feels to lose a mother, and I can't bear the thought that they should have to go through that too soon. I have so many things left to do with them – teach them to drive, shop for prom dresses, plan weddings, be the first to fly with Stephen when he solos, attend the grand opening of Courtney's restaurant. Lord, I pray for time.

May, 2001

…I am so exhausted when I wake, that it's all I can do to drag myself to the medicine cabinet to get that pill. I know that within an hour, I will be able to function. Without it, I feel like I'm going to die. That little pill defines me and rules my life. The kids will soon be home all day, each day of summer and as much as I used to look forward to these months, I've begun to dread them. I will have to make myself get up each day to be with them, since the last thing I want is for them to be home and for me to be in bed.

November, 2001

…I am lonely today for friends, but I am not a good friend to have. At least in my own definition of what a friend should be able to do. Oh, I can be trusted, I can empathize when needed, I don't give advice without it being asked for, and since the age of 27, have not had PMS, so I am rarely moody. But I cannot be depended on to go shopping for hours on end or meet for an occasional lunch. In fact, I've even given up on setting up lunch dates with anyone, because there is nothing worse than having to call a friend and cancel. To cancel once is forgivable, to cancel twice, a bit frustrating but can possibly be understood, but to cancel more than that makes the other person hesitant to do anything with me. And I understand that. So my friends are few and my acquaintances many.

June, 2002
…That stupid medication that was a good thing in the beginning has now become my boss. It took the pain away, but then I started needing the medication just to breathe, just to be able to get out of bed. The doctors and I decided that I needed to get off it, but doing this on my own is ridiculous. I wish we could afford the 5 day treatment, the "rapid detox", but we can't. But I honestly wonder if I'm going to live through this.

September, 2002
…Lord, even my dad is mad at me. Even he doesn't understand, and sits in judgment of me, looking for reasons that aren't there for why I couldn't be there. How I can explain something to him that I don't even understand? I've never felt like I have lived up to his expectations, and being sick was never anything he tolerated, so I must be a huge disappointment to him. I can't take it anymore – this added stress only makes the Lupus worse.

January, 2003
…Tonight was another of those nights that will never be again. Stephen got his first pin during the wrestling match tonight, and I wasn't there to see it. He'll never have a first again. And where was I? Traveling nearly 3 hours each way to go to the only doctor that has been able to actually help me, only to find out that the clinic was closed today, and the trip was fruitless.

Chapter 7

The Wolf wants to eat us all

Over the course of several years dealing with this disease, I had never experienced a flare that lasted so long or one that would require so much attention. I had learned to deal with limping, sitting certain ways, and even holding my arm in such a way that the pain would ease. But instead of living my life managing my illness, I began to let my illness manage me. Not intentionally, of course. Never in a million years would I want to be defined by my illness, but that's exactly what had happened. And once you get to that point, it's incredibly difficult to climb out. That's probably when my family suffered the most. I'll never be able to get those years back, but I can be certain that I will never let this disease steal any more.

The perspectives you are about to read are from my husband and my children. They were very painful for me to read, but very necessary. I want you the reader to understand just how difficult this is not only for me and my family, but for others who have debilitating diseases invading their lives.

Tom's perspective

My wife is my soul mate and God's perfect gift to me. Of all God's blessings to me, she is by far the sweetest. For her I am most grateful, not to mention, I'm crazy about her. She God's beautiful mate for me and a gifted partner in ministry.

I thank God for the faith journey that my family is on. The following is my attempt to put to words some of what this journey with systemic lupus has been the last ten years.

This is very hard to share, since my tendency is to only focus on the positive. But in order to share the true picture of the journey, I must be honest with how it's affected our lives.

I'm so glad that God is daily with us and our battle with lupus. It has been by far the hardest thing for me to deal with in life. On the surface it has robbed us of so many things, suddenly stealing our youthfulness. We have made the decision to let God carry the burden of this chronic illness, but daily it is a struggle to give the anger, fear and disappointment over to him.

It kills me to see my once youthful bride writhing with chronic pain and fatigue, many times unable to leave her bed. Her quality of life is so very poor, many times allowing her to only get out of the house once or twice a week. The pain and fatigue that she wrestles with on a daily basis is off the chart. She hardly ever sleeps due to the excruciating pain of her immune system attacking her chest and connective tissue.

We try to carry on day to day like an average family, making plans with friends or family outings. We are lucky if half of the time those plans can happen as we hope. As a result, we have to cancel, facing disappointment again. This presents a challenge to friendships, as people seem to understand the first few times. But beyond that, we find that many people are simply not up the disappointment. Lupus complicates everything!

The average person struggles to deal with how a week long flu bug disrupts their lifestyle. They simply can not conceive what it's like to live with a chronic illness which stares you in the face every minute of every day. Neither could we if we hadn't experienced first hand ourselves what this is like.

It seems at times that lupus has stolen my wife's youthfulness, cheating her out of the years of a woman's prime time of her life. It's as if she went from her twenties to her seventies, skipping all of the years in between. Her energy level stays so low that it often affects her emotionally. Who wouldn't have a hard time with living life this way? I love her so much and hate to see that in many ways that her youth has been stolen from her. Her health has diminished greatly the last several years. But we know that your strength is proven in our weakness.

The following is an excerpt from one of my journal entries. Journaling helps me to somehow turn these burdens over to God and to better understand.

"God, help us deal with the anger that comes and learn not to direct it towards one another. Help me to help her. Give me wisdom, patience and the ability to be there for Stephen and Courtney as they learn to deal with their mom in bed so much of the time with chronic pain. Give us wisdom as a family to know what activity we can handle and what we can't. And help me to deal with the disappointment of having to cancel plans that we make with others. Please help our church people to understand that if my wife is not able to be in church as she would like to be, that this is simply not possible right now. That we are doing the very best that we can do.

I trust you to free her of the continual fatigue and the pain in her chest and joints. Not to mention the guilt that she carries for not being able to do for her family and for her church as she would like. I trust you each and every day, and I believe that you are completing that healing work in her as each day passes. Until the day in which healing happens, give us the strength and endurance that we need with this debilitating illness. Work your plan to teach us what we need to learn from this and equip us to help others deal with pain in their lives. Help us find a way to give you the ultimate glory for what is going to take place in the future.

Thank you for showing us many things, most importantly for us to be dependent on you. That it is possible to allow the pain that we are in to pull us closer to your side. That we can use whatever pain that we are in to bless other's lives. Teach us the tender compassion of Christ for his people and use us powerfully in the process.

Thank you for the joy of an intimate relationship with Jesus. Teach us to walk more in your spirit and not our own. Teach us to represent Christ wherever we are and to walk in the anointing of your Holy Spirit. Thank you for showing us that freedom in Christ brings the greatest joy, and that serving you is life's greatest honor.

Thank you for teaching us that you are our hope and our only true source, and that we have favor in you. You are our Savior and friend, the supplier of our every need. Thank you for the confidence that we have in you, a confidence that we could never find any place else. It's only by the grace of God that we are over comers and spirit-filled people of faith. In Jesus name, Amen."

Stephen's view

I'm a 17 year old kid getting ready to be a senior next year, so as you probably could imagine, I don't think about anything too deeply, but I'll try. My mom is one of the greatest people I know. She is constantly teaching me about life and how to live it. The hardest thing for me personally is knowing that mom is in pain. I could not imagine what it would be like to live with constant pain. I know when I am sick, I just want everyone to leave me alone and let me stay in my room until I'm better. It amazes me at how positive she is and how she stays in a good mood. There have been times when I have wondered why my mom has lupus. I know there is a reason for everything and maybe it's to help other people cope with their battles, but we may never know. I think my mom having lupus has changed my life, but only in good ways. I think we are all more understanding, compassionate, positive, caring, loving and forgiving because of it.

Courtney's insight

My mom having lupus frustrates me sometimes, mostly because I feel bad that I can't do anything for her. It's hard watching her cringe every time she takes a step because the pain is so horrible. I try to put myself in her position, so I can maybe understand what she goes through. But the truth is I will never know how she feels when she wakes up every day. I know that sometimes she tries to act like she's okay, so we won't worry about her. But most of the time, I see through her. Sometimes I'm angry, not at her, but for not knowing why she can't get better. It tears me up inside. The only thing I know to do is act like it doesn't bother me, when actually it's exactly the opposite. I try to help her by not getting upset when we have to change our plans or something because she doesn't feel up to it. But the truth is, I'm a selfish person, and I do get mad when I've been looking forward to going out for the night, and now we can't because she's hurting and doesn't feel like she can do it. I shouldn't feel that way, and it's something that I'll have to learn to get over. But for now, she has some good days and some bad days, and every day I'm learning more and more about how to deal with the situation. Just because she's sick sometimes, doesn't make her a bad mom. I just hope she knows that I'll love her no matter what, and there's nothing she can do that will change that.

Chapter 8

I'm not the only Red Riding Hood in these woods.

Most people are about as happy as they make up their minds to be.
-- Abraham Lincoln

While doing the research for this book, I first asked the people in my online support group for their stories. I also searched the web for sites committed to personal Lupus narratives. The following is just a short sampling of what I found. The stories have been used with permission.

Sarah's story, age 18

Hi Dene,

I'm glad that you liked my site. When you said the title of your book might be, "but you look so good," I just thought, "I wish I had a nickel for every time that I heard that!"

There are so many people that I don't even want to tell that I have lupus because it seems like you end up being identified by your lupus. I've had lupus for 6 years now, and I'm just getting ready to start college in the spring. So I have no idea how it is going to interfere.

My day-to-day life is basically the same. Throughout the year, my life has to revolve around doctor's appointments and lab tests. From day to day I forget that I have lupus. I can take my pills and not think twice about what they are for. I stay inside all of the time because I'm photosensitive. I don't seem to miss going outside. (I've started to hate the sun.) My lupus doesn't really bother me much because I'm on a lot of medicine. The thing that bothers me the most isn't directly the lupus. The steroids really worked me over. When I was first diagnosed, I was put on a large dose of them and I felt better, but I was starving all of the time, and I almost doubled my weight. So I have stretch marks all over me. Since I've been lowered down on the steroids, I've lost almost 30 pounds in a year and a half. I need to lose another 30 before I'm at my right weight. As you can see, I'm really not all that interesting. But if you want me to elaborate I can.

Take Care,
Sarah

Sarah's story really touched me because even without ever having met her, I could almost sense that she is depressed and lonely. I appreciate her willingness to let me in on a little portion of her life.

Karen's story

Dene,

I was diagnosed with lupus in 1988. And yet even though I don't look sick, it has taken its toll on my body. People cannot see the inside and with lupus, it can attack any organ or muscle. Yes, even the brain. The Lupus caused me to have torn muscles, which put me on social security disability. After trying to survive on the pittance I receive, I decided to try to return to work. I am finding this very hard as it takes all the energy I have just to work 8 hours a day. I'm a true fighter and won't give in. I try to stay in denial all the time until it catches up with me and lands me in the hospital. Lupus runs in my family, I lost my mother and an aunt to lupus, and I have 2 sisters and a niece with lupus. People diagnosed with lupus don't want to have it because there is no cure. I pray one day they will find a cure for lupus, since they can not treat the disease, only the symptoms right now.

Karen D-Brownell

Chris's story

In all my long 47 years of life on this little ball of dirt, I never thought I would have to fight so hard or believe so deeply. The pain, the medications, the doctors and the looks of people who don't understand only make this struggle so much harder. I don't want to be "sick", but my body is genetically made that way.

Actually I am not "sick", but have a chronic condition called Systemic Lupus Erythematosis. It is a condition where my body thinks that it is the enemy and must be defeated. Kind of like the marines fighting against the rest of the armed forces.

In my seven years of searching and diagnosis, I have learned that there is only one lesson to be learned. Life is uncertain. God is a constant. You can never count on life or anyone human to pull you through, but God is always there.

I have been through excruciating pain with no abatement because they couldn't find the right medications, but God held my hand. I have had reactions to the pain killing drugs that made me sicker, but God was by my side. I have bad days and good days, but through it all, God is there by my side to keep me going. I think of Him as my eternal cheerleader. I cannot go a day without His presence.

Don't get me wrong...I have begged and pleaded to be cured and cursed the disease when it didn't go away. We humans have a way of thinking we can do it all and when we can't, thankfully He is there to catch us when we fall.

The hardest part of this whole adventure is the human side. People, even people close to us, don't understand the disease. This disease destroys your life in so many ways. The fatigue is so deep that at times, just breathing is a chore. Blinking your eyelids is like walking the Sahara desert. The pain is on the inside, so there are days when you want a Morphine drip, but on the outside you look great! Someone who doesn't understand will come along and tell you how great you look, and you start to feel sorry for yourself and start falling into that pit of despair.

After seven years I have eliminated all the insensitive people in my life. People who don't understand that I can't stay out until midnight or I will hurt the next day, have just wandered off and not returned. People I have known for years don't even acknowledge that I exist anymore, and I have changed churches to avoid the constant tension. LUPUS IS NOT CONTAGIOUS, but you would think it was. Family avoid me because I can no longer drop everything and help them dig or plant or paint. It is just too hard for my bones and muscles to do such work.

I am not lazy...I just hurt so badly, most days that I can barely walk.

To anyone who reads this.... get information and stop looking at the outside. God doesn't look at the outside.... only the inside. Look at the heart, because that is where God resides.

Chris

A father's perspective

I will never forget that phone call 9 years ago. It was from my daughter, Debbie, who lived in California. "Daddy," she said, "they just diagnosed what's wrong with me. The doctor said I have systemic lupus erythematosus." - she could hardly pronounce the disease, no less understand what she, at 21 years of age, was about to face for a long time.

The words struck me like an arrow. Systemic lupus something or other. What was it? I never

heard of this disease. I felt completely ignorant, helpless, afraid and alone. What did I do or not do to bring this disease on - this disease that neither of us could pronounce nor understand?

"Debbie," I said, "don't worry, I'll find out all I can about it and get back to you." That's all I could say at the moment - the most important moment in my daughter's life and all her educated, all knowing, loving father could say was I'll get back to you with some answers. What answers - was there a cure - was it life threatening - how much pain will she have to endure - what kind of life will she now

lead - how can we as parents help her - should she move back to New Jersey - should we move to California - on and on these questions ran through my head.

All of a sudden I felt great anger gripping my body. Why my beautiful daughter - why her in the early stages of her life - why her, who loves life so much and has so much to live for. Why have you done this to her? The you I still cannot figure out.

How did a loving father cope these past 9 years? How do all you parents, spouses, siblings - significant others who have loved ones afflicted with lupus - cope? How do you deal with anger, guilt, fear and so many feelings mixed up inside of you everyday as you see your loved one suffer? When you want to take the pain away and cannot. When you want to say, "give it to me, let me suffer with it so you may go on and live a normal life."

I, like may of you, have found some answers and a great deal of support from the Lupus Foundation. In my case, the Lupus Foundation of New Jersey provided that support. I first joined for very selfish reasons. I wanted knowledge, information I could pass on to my daughter and to help me understand what this disease was all about. What effect will drugs have on her body? Are there alternate treatments? What about nutrition, diet, exercise, etc., etc., etc.? I asked many, many questions, attended many meetings, spoke with many doctors and got some answers, not enough - there had to be some other way. It was then I decided thebest source of information, the best way I as a parent could cope with this disease was to get involved directly with lupus patients. Get to know them, them to know me - what it feels like being a parent. To put to work my skills as a trained "Behavioral Counselor" to help them and they help me.

I began conducting rap groups, support groups for patients and significant others. I've learned more about the disease, as well as how to cope more effectively as a parent from those sessions than from all the medical lectures I've attended. I found the answers to many questions - the answer that in most cases you, the lupus patient, have more knowledge about the disease and its affect on your body than any physician. That each one of you must become more assertive and forthright concerning the treatment you favor. That the most important aspect of the doctor-patient relationship is that your doctor be a good listener, as well as someone you can depend on.

In turn I've shared my knowledge concerning the importance of a positive self-concept and feeling good about oneself in coping with lupus, of how to deal more effectively with stress and the impact of "mind on the body."

We've learned from each other, we laugh, cry, share feelings, touch each other and together me, a parent, and they, the patient learning from it, deals more effectively with his feelings, as well as being able to communicate with his daughter. In summary, I am calling on all of you out there - all you parents, spouses, significant others - get involved - no more feelings of loneliness, no more feelings of helplessness, of guilt. We need each other, we need all the human resources we can mobilize in the fight against lupus - we must give our loved ones the message - you are not alone - you will never be alone - we are as one.

Chapter 9

Thorns in the thicket

Stand up to crises. Don't let them throw you! Fight to stay calm...even surmount the crisis completely and turn it into an opportunity. Refuse to renounce your self-image. No matter what happens, you must keep your good opinion of yourself. No matter what happens, you must hold your past successes in your imagination, ready for showing in the motion picture screen of your mind. No matter what happens, no matter what you lose, no matter what failures you must endure, you must keep faith in yourself. Then you can stand up to crises, with calm and courage, refusing to buckle; then you will not fall through the floor. You will be able to support yourself.

Insurance is a thorn in my side, and is one of the most frustrating parts of this disease. In order to get great care and actually benefit from your insurance, you must never get sick, and you must stay healthy. May God help you if you ever are without insurance! Without insurance, you have no choice but to either do without medical care, which I have done for years, which causes greater harm to me and inevitably makes the disease worse, which in turn shortens my life, which in turn makes the time I have here almost unbearable sometimes. Or, you can pay for all the care out of pocket, which we have also done. That has caused us to not be able to save for our future, among other things.

My prescriptions alone are over $600 a month, not to mention the constant need for extensive testing. The average Lupus patient should expect to spend at least $12,000 a year to stay on top of the disease. But if you don't have insurance, that money has to come from someplace, or you do like many, including myself, and simply go without care. Then when the money runs out and the husband has to take on two or three extra jobs to be able to have more money to care for you, and you are already about as low as you think you can go, you have to tuck your tail between your legs and ask for assistance. First you apply for Disability, which is virtually impossible to get, not to mention an agency that even admits in the workbook they provide to aid people in the process of filing, that most, if not all claims, are first reviewed (and I use that term loosely) by untrained, uneducated office workers, who do nothing but open envelopes and stamp DENIED across the front. Then you tuck your tail even further between your legs and reapply, only to be denied again. It is common knowledge that you will be rejected twice before your application is ever considered. In the meantime, you have to have meds and have to see doctors, but have no money to do it, so you wrap your tail around your head and seek public assistance, which is, literally, the bottom of the barrel.

The best and worst part of this process has been the lessons learned while on Medicaid. After the initial shame sets in, once you've realized you have nowhere else to go, no more resources to tap, the humiliation is quick to follow. We applied for Medicaid just for me, since my medical needs and expenses were going to be more than we could afford. It was just during the few months my husband was between jobs. Without medical attention, my disease was sure to get worse, and since I had been struggling for almost two years already with a terrible flare involving my lungs, we had to do something, even if it meant humiliation.

Keep in mind, we were the average American 2 kids, 2 cars middle-income family. We had excellent credit, a mortgage we had never missed a payment on, a couple of credit cards and enough money in the bank to last us about 3 months if we were ever in a pinch. We were not rich, and we were not poor. We knew the value of money and bought the best quality we could afford, and then we made it last by taking very good care of it.

Being in ministry for over 15 years, we had to economize, but that never meant that what we had couldn't look nice. God gave me the gift of frugality matched with a decorator's eye, and I've been known to turn a lot of other people's trash into magnificent treasures with nothing more that a can of paint. To the outside world, we were often judged incorrectly as being rich when indeed we have simply been blessed. Long story short, we could comfortably mingle with stock market executives, bank presidents, and fit in well in most country club environments, without the six-figure income needed to maintain those lifestyles.

Plus we had history on our side. Both of us had come from a long line of hard working family members who had impeccable work ethics, so we had no familiarity with The System or anyone who knew how to work it. We had not been socially brainwashed into believing that public assistance was an inevitable part of our lives and our children's futures. It was like learning about a lifestyle and culture we knew nothing about.

The following is a journal entry I wrote while waiting to see a doctor at a free clinic.

I am sitting in a free clinic, and my initial feelings are embarrassment. I used to feel this way when I would take my mother to see her cancer specialist. My mouth wanted to cry out explanations, letting them know that I wasn't one of "them". But my mother never seemed to notice the "looks," she didn't seem to be embarrassed at all. And she needn't have been. She hadn't chosen her circumstances, much like I haven't chosen mine. So, if she had no reason to feel shame, why should I?

Maybe I wouldn't feel this way as much, if I hadn't been treated like trash. Treated like I was a product of the legacy of poverty, which to the world equaled ignorance, filth and stupidity, just to name a few. And wasn't I guilty of dishing out those judgments? How else would I know so much about what other people were thinking?

I am beginning to be comfortable here in this waiting room, listening to conversations of women so very different from me and yet just like me. Lupus is our common denominator.

Frustration! Oh my, I'm so tired of being frustrated. Frustrated first because the doctor I was seeing treated the symptoms, not the disease. Secondly, frustrated with doctors who talk down to me for whatever reason – either because I'm on Medicaid and that's how people in my position are supposed to be treated, or simply because she's a "Dr." and I'm not. I'm frustrated with myself because I don't understand their medical language. All I want is a doctor who will listen, understand, empathize and answer my questions, without making me feel as if I'm ignorant for asking, stupid for not understanding "the system" and ashamed of myself for being on assistance. The last visit here with Dr. James was so enlightening and encouraging, and most importantly, hopeful. Now today is just the opposite. No answers, no hope. What was determined last time as "typically Lupus" is today not Lupus at all. Two doctors, two opinions, same office. If I didn't feel so bad, I would just curl up and quit. I give up.

They want me to have a general practitioner, a family doctor, but don't understand how limited our choices are, and besides who wants to see a doctor who prescribes valium and who's staff treats me like trash? And he is the best choice as far as doctors who accept Medicaid in Muskogee. On one occasion, I waited 4 hours to be seen, and became aware that the people waiting with me had appointment times after mine and were getting in before me simply because they had "real" insurance. Apparently, when I questioned the receptionist, I was told that I would be seen only after the paying patients had all been seen. That alone was humiliating enough, but once inside the examining room, the physician's nurse asked me some questions pertaining to my medication history, seeming to size me up and judge me because I had been on a very strong narcotic and was now asking for something to help me sleep. I could tell by her tone that she did not approve, and I began to feel like the child who is in trouble, as if I had done something wrong. If that wasn't bad enough, she took it one step farther and used the term "drug-seeking" in her description of me, and that's when I walked out.

No wonder people who have to be part of the system, either because they are born into it, or because of poor choices, or like me, was left with no choice if I wanted any medical care at all, get stuck in the system. It doesn't take long to start believing you are the scum of the earth, when that's how you are treated on a regular basis.

Lord, please don't ever let me think that I am better than anyone else.

Chapter 10

The Wolf wore Grannie's clothes

Many are the plans in a man's heart, but it is the Lord's purpose that prevails. -- Proverbs 19:21

Red Riding Hood didn't expect the Wolf to outsmart her and use the information she had given him to beat her to Grannie's house. Upon hearing that Grannie may be ailing, she does what her mother asks of her. Her plans were simple – deliver the basket of goodies to Grannie, have a nice visit, and then skip all the way home. But the unexpected meeting with Mr. Wolf changed all that.

My life wasn't going as I planned it either. When Tom and I got married, I had a specific vision of how things would unfold. We would have 2 or 3 children, and I would stay home to raise and nurture until they were old enough to be in school. Then the plan was to begin a career or go back to school, knowing we would need the extra income. Most importantly, I wanted to be an active mother. I wanted to be the homeroom mom that organized seasonal parties. To be able to eat lunch in the cafeteria on a weekly basis, ride bikes and shop were just basic expectations. But about the time that I was about to realize my vision, Lupus entered the picture. All the basic expectations, not to mention the entire vision, had been tossed out the window.

Gone was the notion of being in charge of class parties for fear I would no longer be able to be counted on. Riding bikes together would rarely happen because the pain from my feet and legs didn't allow it and the incredible fatigue could keep me in bed for days afterward. Suddenly the plan for my life, my plan that is, had changed. Not only had I planned on being an active mother and wife, but I had plans to be an active ministry partner with my husband. Now the word "active" had been thrown out of my vocabulary. All of a sudden, my plans were changed. I have a little bit of an obsessive compulsive personality, and I don't handle change well. Facing the uncertainty of what lay ahead of me in my future was extremely frustrating.

This disease started costing me right from the beginning. During the first couple of years, I continued life as usual, but since stress is a huge factor in the disease, after a few busy days and lots of activity, my mind and my body would crash. But it wasn't my job or church that paid the price, it was my family. I'm a people pleaser, and at the time, I spent so much time trying to keep everyone happy, that I completely overlooked the needs of my family. Many, many evenings, we would plan to go out to dinner as a family, or maybe just take a walk, and I couldn't go. The kids certainly didn't understand; how could they when Tom and I didn't understand, and then the added guilt from upsetting the plans just burdened me more.

Within two years of my diagnosis, I had to quit my job. I was working as a secretary for one of the schools and was using at least 3 sick days a month. We really needed the income, since we had just built a new home, but my health just wouldn't permit it. I didn't know it at the time, but I was slowly beginning the process of realizing that I couldn't do it all. Up until then, I was determined that I could still pursue the plans I had made for my life and manage a chronic illness at the same time.

Chapter 11

Woodcutters to the Rescue

Every day holds the possibility of a miracle. – Unknown

Over the course of nearly a decade, this illness has cost me dearly, in more ways than I care to remember. Not only has it cost me, but it has cost my family as well. Sometimes it has cost me resentment from extended family members who don't understand why I can't be at a family event or church members who don't understand why I'm unable to be at every event. But family is family, and in spite of our situation, they continue to love unconditionally. Unfortunately, I can't say the same about people who have called themselves my friends. Losing friendships or just not being able to cultivate new ones has been a significant cost in this journey. And it's not all their fault, it's mine as well. Having already lost many and not being able to live up to the expectations of a participating member of a friendship, I tend to hold back, not wanting to get hurt again, not wanting to be a disappointment. Of course it doesn't help that I have a huge phone phobia. The internet has become a great source of communication for me though, thank goodness.

Not having an abundance of close friends is fine, since I have a huge assortment of acquaintances and extended family. There is no downside to that, since it causes me to truly value the real friends I have. Those are the friends who stick by me no matter what, no matter how many times I can't make a lunch engagement, no matter how many times I have to cancel plans, no matter how many times I'm unable to return a phone call. Friends like that are hard to come by, especially the older I get, but I am blessed to say that God has given me more true friends in this new millennium than I have ever had.

I also have made faceless friends on the internet through an internet Lupus support group. One of those friends had the most impact on me and this situation than anyone has ever made. Support groups are opportunities for support, obviously, but they also provide a forum for laughter, camaraderie, and for me, a place to vent about my frustration with the plans I had made for my life that I was unable to fulfill thanks to Lupus. But I was so fortunate to come across a very wise woman in that support group, and something she said to me became the turning point, the catalyst to who I am now, not who I was. She has listened through our correspondence to me whine and bellyache about how having Lupus was not in the plans I had for my life, that I had gifts that God had given me, and now, thanks to Lupus, all those gifts and all those plans could never be. She had probably heard enough, but very wisely andvery gently, she told me that I had to grieve the person I used to be, that I had to let her go and celebrate the person I am now. She reminded me that I still have value, that if I don't embrace the person I am with Lupus, that no one else would either. Such wisdom!

The first and most difficult process was the grieving. It was very similar to the way I felt when my mother died. I had to stop living in the past, stop feeling guilty for what I had missed. I had to believe that I was still a good mother, a good wife and a whole person with Lupus. It was so painful, and just like when my mother died, I had to stop playing the "if only" game. I had to quit blaming myself, quit believing that somehow I had done something to deserve this.

And just like the death of a loved one, the grief is ongoing. Several times while writing this book, I've had to get up from the computer and walk away, the reality of the words I was writing was more than I could bear. Sometimes I had to cry, to mourn again for what was lost and would never be. But I realize that with or without Lupus, life goes on, and we all know just how quickly it passes.

The acceptance came next. Acceptance of the way things are now and the courage to go on. God gave me a very real picture of what my life is and how to make the best use of my gifts during my quiet time with Him one day. I was looking around me at the beautiful things we had acquired over the years. Some were cherished family heirlooms that had been passed down to me, many were gifts we had received, and I noticed how over time, each one had found a place to rest, a purpose to serve. I was thinking about our first home and the meager furnishings we had. My gaze stopped at a crystal vase that had been a wedding gift many years ago, and I remembered that when we were first married, as much as I loved the gift, I had no place for it. It didn't really fit into our "décor" if you could call it that, our mismatched, combined furnishings, leftover from college days, style. But even though it had no real purpose at the time, I certainly didn't get rid of it, instead I put it aside to use later. I certainly didn't get angry because I couldn't use it, I just carefully wrapped it up and packed it away, knowing that eventually it would have a place. And now, after almost 20 years, it fit into collection of beautiful pieces, and I was so thankful that I still had it. In fact, I think I value it more now, remembering how I had taken great care to see to it that it wouldn't get broken during our many moves, and more importantly, it had become a sentimental piece now, not one of monetary value. The person who had given it to us had gone on to be with Jesus, making it even more valuable to me as a reminder of the love that person had for us.

And then it dawned on me that the gifts that God had given me still had a place in my life. Maybe not the way I had originally intended, but it didn't matter, because 20 years ago I didn't really grasp the value of the gift. Maybe I wouldn't have used those gifts the way God intended me to, and maybe He had allowed me to grow and mature during this journey so that I would fully appreciate the gift and the Giver.

So I'm not famous Broadway star or a Nobel Peace Prize winner. My figure is not what it used to be and I've added a multitude of wrinkles to my face. And that's okay. God loves me just the way I am.

If I have to count the cost of living with Lupus, of coming face to face with the Wolf, I would say the cost has been great, but I think it has made me better because of it. Sometimes we don't understand why we have to walk through life's path with a thorn in our side, but that's because we can't see the roses blooming behind us.

Chapter 12

The Fairy Tale Ends, Life Begins

for all that You've done I will thank you,
for all that You're going to do,
for all that You've promised and all that You are
is all that has carried me through
Jesus I thank You
    Dennis Jernigan, "Thank You, Lord", Giant Killer Album

Be glad for all God is planning for you. Be patient...and prayerful always. -- Romans 12:12 TLB

Thus I will bless You while I live; I will lift up my hands in Your name. My soul shall be satisfied as with marrow and fatness, and my mouth shall praise You with joyful lips.
*   Psalm 63:4-5*

Today I am still living with Lupus, but I face each day with a better attitude, and if the day doesn't turn out to be the way I hoped, if I have pain that I didn't expect, I know that there is always tomorrow. I try to use the pain as a reminder of the agony that was suffered on my behalf, all those years ago on the cross. I am thankful that it is me with the pain, and not my husband or my children, because I could not bear it.

And I am not perfect, but a work in process. I do not always handle the pain like I should, and sometimes I get angry. I take out my frustration on the ones closest to me, and then have to ask for their forgiveness. When I have those moments or days, it is usually because I'm trying to do it alone. I'm trying to carry the burden by myself, and those times I fail are reminders that I don't have to do this without God. I am reminded just how fortunate I am that I have Someone who wants to carry this burden for me, and I shift the load from my shoulders to His.

Hope is what keeps me going. Hope that one day I may not have Lupus or that the doctors will find a cure. Miracles happen all the time, and I never stop asking. But until then, I'm going to be the best person I can be and find something to smile about.

Above my front door I have a vine of dried honeysuckle wrapped in greenery. Over the course of time it has been there, several birds have decided to call it home. On days when it was difficult to do much more than brush my teeth, I would make it a goal to go to the door and watch the birds. Each and every day they worked. They picked up every stick and leaf and piece of straw they could find to build their nest, their home, usually in preparation for the birth of the baby birds. Living in Oklahoma, or tornado alley, I knew that at some point the wind was going to blow so hard that their nest would be destroyed and maybe even their little family would be lost in the storms that came every spring. And they may have known it, too. But it never stopped them from working, preparing and planning.

One morning after a particularly windy, stormy night, I walked to the door and saw that the honeysuckle garland had been blown down, and their nest was gone. As I stood there, feeling sad for them, I heard a sweet sound coming from the porch. Their home may have been destroyed and their family lost, *but it didn't stop them from singing.* In spite of what they had experienced, in spite of the pain, they still found something to sing about.

My mother battled ovarian cancer for 8 months before she went to live with Jesus. During that entire 8 months, not once did she ever feel sorry for herself, not once did she ever ask why, not once did she ever get angry. In fact, she was almost too happy. She was so happy sometimes, that people forgot she was sick. She spent every day investing in everyone else, trying to make them feel better. She kept a journal during that time, and in not one entry does she complain or seem troubled about the journey she was on. She used the energy that she had, which at times was little to none, to pray for those around her, to send cards to strangers and write silly poems. My mother didn't live a wonderful life; in fact, she had lived most of her life in a way that wasn't pleasing to God or her family. Because of some poor choices she had made, she had very little when it came to worldly possessions, and really, little to show for a life spanning over 50 years. Up until a couple of years before her cancer diagnosis, she and I had little to do with one another, and I had few, if any, fond memories of her.

But when God gave us the opportunity to share the last 8 months of her life together, she didn't spend that time feeling sorry for herself and making everyone around her miserable. She didn't spend the money she had on possessions she had always wanted. She knew her days were numbered, and she chose instead to use that time to leave a mark, a legacy. I didn't realize it at the time, in fact, much of the time I resented having to take care of her when she had never been a mother to me. Because she had no insurance and was on public assistance, I also watched as various medical doctors and nurses treated her with little, to no, respect. But she seemed oblivious to it, and smiled and was nicer to them than they deserved. She laughed. She gave compliments. Nothing could get her down, nothing could steal her joy, even with the knowledge that she knew she would die, and she knew it would be a painful death. She never gave in to it, and she found the good and God in every situation, all the way to the end.

If you've never been with someone right before they die, you've really missed a blessing. Mother Theresa once said that being with those who are dying is as close as you get in this life to being with God himself. When someone is dying, they aren't asking for material possessions, they aren't concerned about their appearance; all that matters to them is being with the ones they love.

The night before my mother died, I had been with her at the hospital for several days and nights without much sleep. We didn't know how much longer she had, but my husband and I agreed that I needed to go home and rest for at least one night. She had stopped talking several hours before and could only communicate with her eyes. I looked at her before I left, and told her that if the angels came while I was gone, that she should go with them. I hugged her and walked out the door, and she died a few hours later, while I was home, asleep.

I felt terrible guilt for a long time that I hadn't been there when she went with the angels. But it dawned on me later that even as she died, she had been looking out for me. I really believe that she didn't want me to have the memory of what may have happened as her body shut down as my last memory of her. She was making my life better, even in death.

That's what I want for my kids. Not that I'm going to die soon, I certainly plan on being around long enough to spoil some grandchildren and maybe even some great grandchildren. But I want to make sure that the last memory I leave with my family every day is a good one, and that the legacy I'm creating is a pleasant one, one they can look back and smile and laugh about.

I believe we should approach every day as if it's our last. Death is the one certainty that will come knocking on all our doors, we just don't know when. No matter what lies ahead; be it getting wrinkles, losing my hair or even great pain, whatever it is, I don't ever want to stop enjoying life and being with the people I love. I want to make sure that the people I love always know just how special they are to me, how much they mean. I want to make sure I take the time to tell them the things I sometimes think, but am afraid to say for fear it may sound mushy and embarrass them. I want the joy life gives me to spill over so much that it overshadows anything else they may see when they look at me. I want to spread that joy so that when people are around me they feel good, not because *of* me, but because of what's *in* me - of *Who* is in me.

I imagine that little Red Riding-Hood pulled her hood over her curls and set off down the sunny green slope, with her basket in her hand, at a brisk pace. But as she got deeper into the forest, she walked more slowly. Everything was so beautiful; the great trees waved their huge arms over her, the birds were calling to one another from the thorns all white with blossom, and the child began singing as she went. She could not have told why, but I think it was because the beauty around her made her feel glad. She never expected her path to cross with the Wolf.

Just when she thought that the wolf was about to have her for dessert, two tall wood-cutters rushed in with their heavy axes and killed the wicked Wolf in far less time that it takes to tell you about it.

"But where is Grannie?" asked Little Red Riding-Hood, when she had thanked the brave wood-cutters. "Oh! Where can poor Grannie be? Can the cruel Wolf have eaten her up?"

And she began to cry and sob bitterly - when, who should walk in but Grannie herself, as large as life, and as hearty as ever, with her marketing-basket on her arm! For it was another old dame in the village who was not very well, and Grannie had been down to visit her and give her some of her own famous herb-tea.

So everything turned out right in the end, and all lived happily every after.

Lord, I don't ever want to stop singing, no matter what. And never, never again, will I be afraid of the big, bad wolf.

We have been given yesterdays for a reason
They were meant to be filled with memories
We cannot count tomorrows
But we can count yesterdays
And most importantly
We can make today count

Dene' Hopkins